Principles Of Exercise

Your Ideal Body

Table of Contents

Copyright ©2017, Oswin Dacosta

These are some of my other books below, and my website is
www.LosingBellyFatMission.com :

https://www.amazon.com/dp/B06XB4WHZX http://www.amazon.com/dp/B06X9LXBB8
http://www.amazon.com/dp/B06WLK7497

http://www.amazon.com/dp/B06W54JKQN http://www.amazon.com/dp/B06X6DJ9K3
http://www.amazon.com/dp/B06WGNJ9N3 http://www.amazon.com/dp/B06W549TBD
http://www.amazon.com/dp/B06VTF5DQJ http://www.amazon.com/dp/B06WRPSBKK
http://www.amazon.com/dp/B06WD194JR http://www.amazon.com/dp/B06WCZTK7Y
http://www.amazon.com/dp/B06X3QN1HT http://www.amazon.com/dp/B01N19WBF2
http://www.amazon.com/dp/B01N2AVECA http://www.amazon.com/dp/B01N4VZIAV
http://www.amazon.com/dp/B00QJJFS1C http://www.amazon.com/dp/B01EMNO2MW
http://www.amazon.com/dp/B00SSFWCPA http://www.amazon.com/dp/1520531230
http://www.amazon.com/dp/B01N4V7SR9 http://www.amazon.com/dp/B00SX58DUI
http://www.amazon.com/dp/B010K7YP62 http://www.amazon.com/dp/B012LAYNNQ
http://www.amazon.com/dp/B00RVX3KY2 http://www.amazon.com/dp/B01MR6SWGW
http://www.amazon.com/dp/B00XF6G4HO http://www.amazon.com/dp/B01F1472N2
http://www.amazon.com/dp/B00PQ0TUPU http://www.amazon.com/dp/B00PP8OZJ4
http://www.amazon.com/dp/B00QH7DY4Y http://www.amazon.com/dp/B01052010G
http://www.amazon.com/dp/B00QDHXN7Q http://www.amazon.com/dp/B00PO0IQIO

Among others.

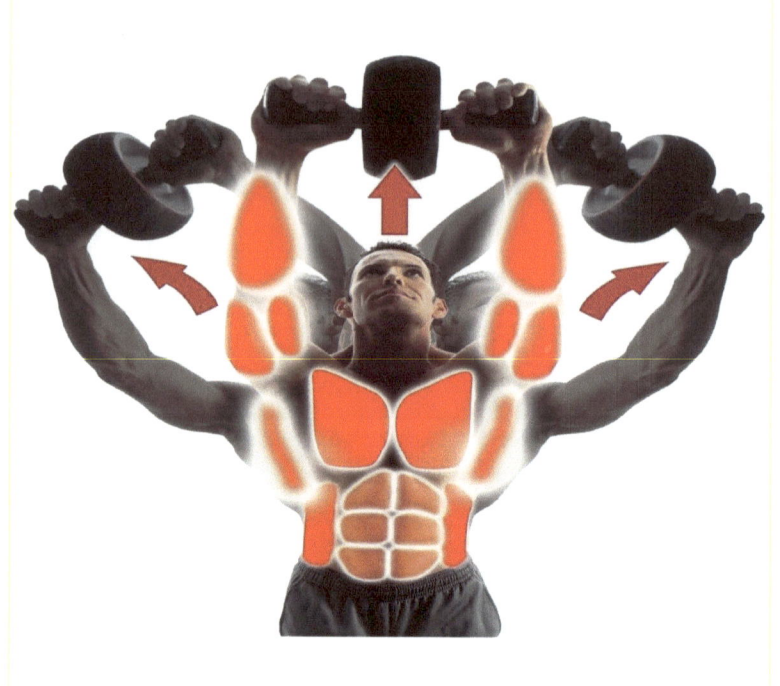

Exercise, or regular exercise, is not just a fad that you can go in and out of anytime you want. Exercise is something that needs to be done with dedication and perseverance. There are some things that a beginner should know about exercise, whether they are into losing weight, cardio exercises, or bodybuilding. Here are some of the basic principles of exercise that everyone should know.

Recent studies show that it is better to exercise during the afternoon rather than in the morning. This time of day is where your body's energy level is at its peak. In the morning, your energy level is comparably low. However, there is a traditional belief that starting your day with exercise will make you feel more alive all throughout the day. The old belief is also true, but exercising in the afternoon spares you more energy to endure the morning's activities.

Another basic principle in exercise is that you cannot rush the effects of exercise on your body. If you double the load or spend more time working out than you should, you will only become prone to what others call exercise burnout. To avoid this, you need to build up a pace gradually. If you are into lifting weights, start with a lighter load. If you are into cardio exercises, start with shorter sessions.

Never try to speed up or double the time for a routine as this may cause more disadvantages than benefits. Remember, exercise burnout happens if you want to reach your goal in shorter periods of time than what is realistic for you to accomplish it.

Finally, the most important principle in exercise is never to lay off your schedule unless something really important comes up. You may need to have a very flexible schedule in case you have a job that needs immediate attention. For most professionals, having home fitness equipment is always a big help. Even when they come home late from work, they still could sneak 30 minutes or so for exercise because they have their own home fitness equipment. Even if you have no time to do it at the gym, you could do your exercise at home if you have a treadmill or an elliptical trainer. These are just three of the most helpful principles that every person should follow when they workout.

To sum it all up, it is better to exercise in the afternoon, don't rush when you exercise, and never try to ditch off the exercise schedule that you started so you would achieve the goal that you have set. Even if you have achieved your weight loss or fat loss goals, you surely have found out for yourself that maintenance of your new healthy weight takes consistent effort as well. Keep these exercise tips in mind and you'll do just fine.

Facts About Getting A Flatter Stomach

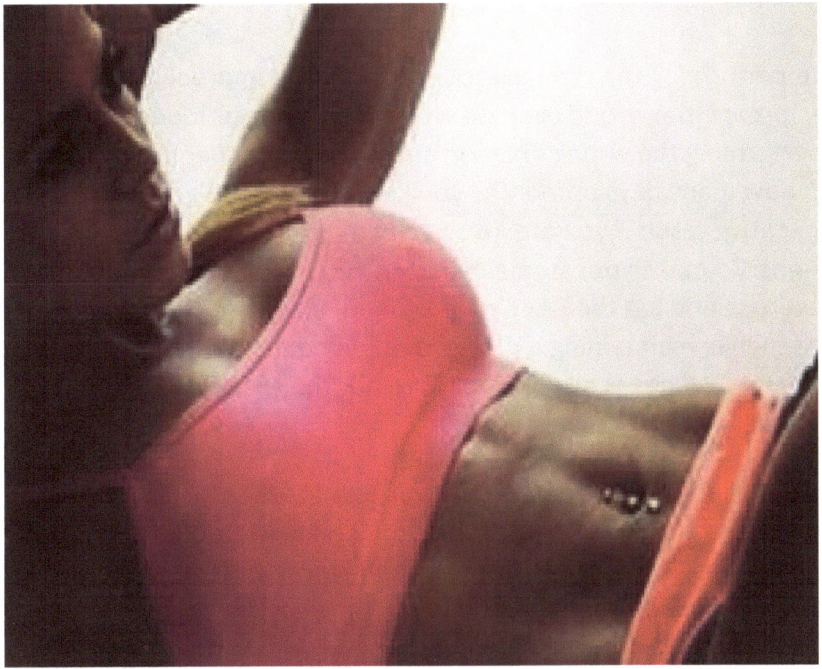

Women are so focused and preoccupied with ideas in working out to obtain a flatter stomach. Several of them are trapped with misconceptions about doing heavy work outs in the gym or tiring exercises at home. And while doing these, they never are worried eating whatever they want. They will only tell you that extra calories are after all burned during the exercise. Obviously if you continue doing this, you will surely wonder why after a few months your stomach still is the same. You for sure will be asking yourself what could have been wrong with your exercise that everything resulted to nothing. Still, you did not achieve what you have expected. To give you a clear explanation, here are three possible causes why you keep on failing in obtaining a flatter stomach despite the heavy exercises you did.

You are performing the right exercise while eating improper foods. You are performing the wrong exercise while eating proper foods. You are both performing the wrong exercise and eating improper foods. No matter how many days or months you keep on exercising, you will still get a negative result if you are involved with any of these three conditions. To make your stomach flatter, you have to perform the right exercise and eat the right kinds of food. If you are doing the right exercises while maintaining a proper diet, no doubt you can reach your goal. Doing crunches or sit-ups really are not the exercises for stomach. All these are just part of the myth.

The real or practical way of flattening your stomach is actually through cardio exercises. Two of the most common types of cardio exercises are jogging and walking. For 20 to 40 minutes, you can jog or walk. If you want to have a little fun while doing the exercise, you can enjoy cycling around the park. But if don't want to go outside, you can do a cardio exercise at home by using the jumping rope. If you have Wii, you can even make it more enjoyable by playing boxing or tennis with using your Wii. You can actually make exercises for stomach pleasurable and entertaining.

The main point of cardio exercises is actually to raise your heart rate. Any form of exercise where you can start to feel that your heart rate is increasing, you essentially boost your metabolism. Burning down your cholesterol and fats especially stomach fats is the main target of cardio exercises. This form of flat stomach exercise should be done at least three times a week or best you do it daily. If you are new to exercising, do not immediately begin in a fast pace. You might distress your body if you do this; always keep in mind to begin in a slower pace. If you are unsure about what you are doing, you can purchase CDs, DVDs, magazines or books which can give you the right guides and tips for a proper exercise and a proper diet.

These resources will reveal you the secret when it comes to the real flat stomach exercise. As long as you have the determination and the passion, you can definitely get a flatter and sexier stomach!

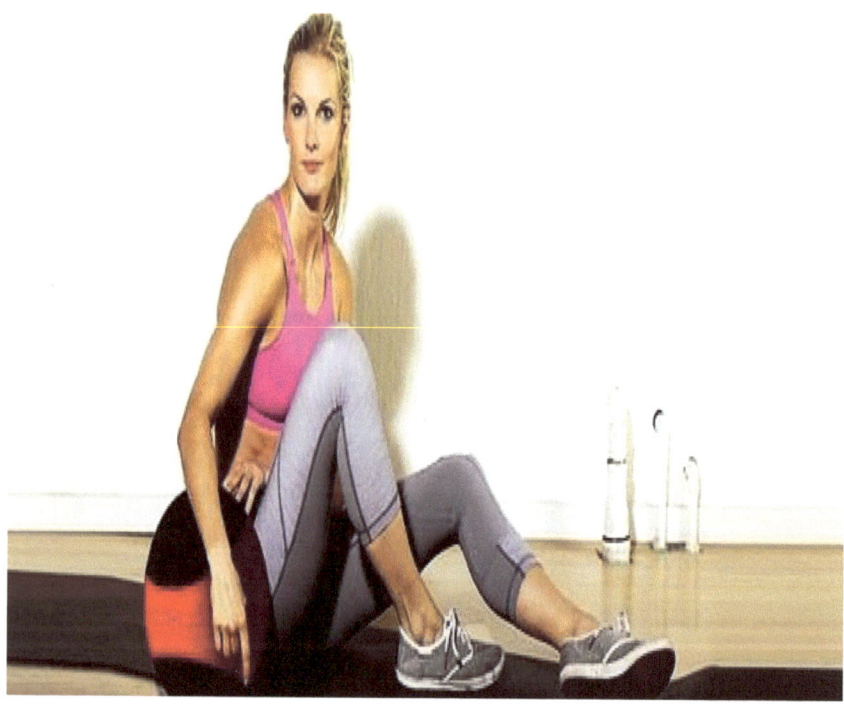

Being obese is no joke. This is a life threatening condition that could ultimately lead to others. You have to find a way to reach your body's ideal weight and stay there is you want to avoid these health conditions. In this article you will find ways on how you can maintain your weight.

#1 Find out what your body mass index is. To get this number you divide your weight in kilograms by your height in meters and then divide that number by your height in meters again. If your number comes out to be more than 25, you are considered overweight.

#2 When exercising, start slow and progress. Try biking, jogging, swimming or brisk walking for at least 30 minutes a day in order to sweat and get your heart pumping. A walk around the neighborhood or in the park doesn't necessarily count as exercise.

#3 Don't limit yourself to cardio exercises. The way to build muscle and stamina is to do more intense weight training and interval training than cardio. Just use the cardio exercises for a warm up so that you will get better results.

#4 Eat less, but more frequently. Eat six or more small meals per day it is better than having three big meals. When you space out a few small meals per day, you keep your metabolism going which burns more calories and prevents more fat from building.

If you were to follow these few simple healthy tips to get to and stay at your ideal weight, you will be successful. You can also take it a step further by taking meal supplements, choosing healthier meal alternatives and increase the intensity level of your workout routines. You can also pay a quick visit to your doctor if you still have questions regarding anything we discussed here today.

Get Fit With Cardiovascular Exercise

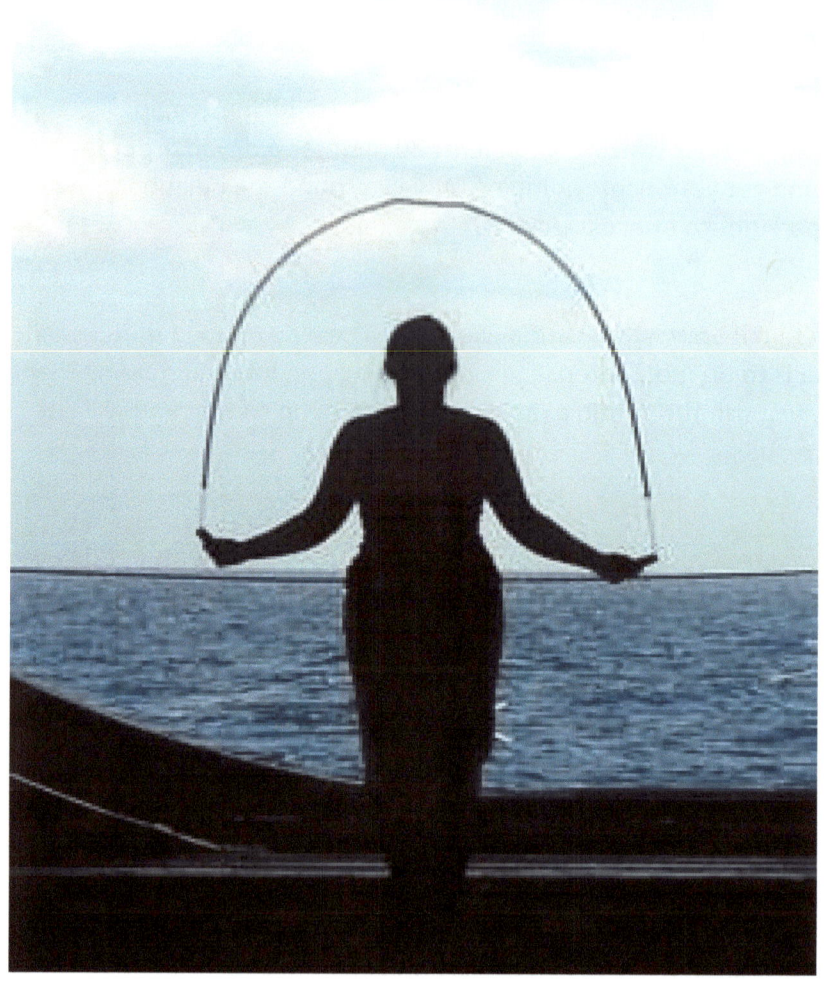

The general rule about weight loss is simple - no pain, no gain! But flattening your belly and forgetting about love handles doesn't necessarily mean giving up on flavorful and delicious food. Only 15% less calories, combined with intensive cardio training can create miracles. Cardio exercises are the essence of every efficient weight loss program. They help you burn fat and improve health at the same time.

Cardio training doesn't have to be strenuous and devastating - you can do aerobic workouts without completely draining your energy. Try cycling, slow running or brisk walking instead of treadmills, steppers and elliptical machines at the local gym to make it even more enjoyable.

You can also jump the rope, swim or walk the stairs anywhere - as long as your heartbeat rate is increased for a long or extended period of time. The right intensity of cardio training is should get you to 120-140 heartbeats per minute.

There are also a couple of more rules - try exercising in the morning, with your stomach still empty, because your body burns fat reserves instead of a freshly eaten meal. In order to start the fat burning process, you need at least 30 minutes of exercise, because in the first 20 minutes, your body uses sugar reserves in your muscles instead of fat. So, choose the exercise and place (although walking is the preferred weight loss method for obese people) and bear in mind the timetable in the first 12 minutes, your body uses the sugar which you already have stored in the muscles. From 12th to 20th minute, you are using reserves which are easy to re-build. From 30th to 60th minute, you are using those fatty reserves, the ones you wanted to get rid of in the first place! After 60 minutes, your body is very tired, and tries to keep all of the reserves. The risk of injury grows with every minute after.

For longer trainings, you really need persistence and great motivation. Be ready to follow your goals to the very end and make yourself proud. Get that fancy dress or beautiful suit out you dreamed of wearing for a very long time and enjoy your new life as a slimmer and healthier person, just like those lucky people whom you envied only a couple of months before. Be ready to embrace the challenge of a lifetime and do cardio by walking anywhere you want - in shops, in malls, downtown or in parks - it's completely up to you. Just do it with your head held high and keep your goals always in sight.

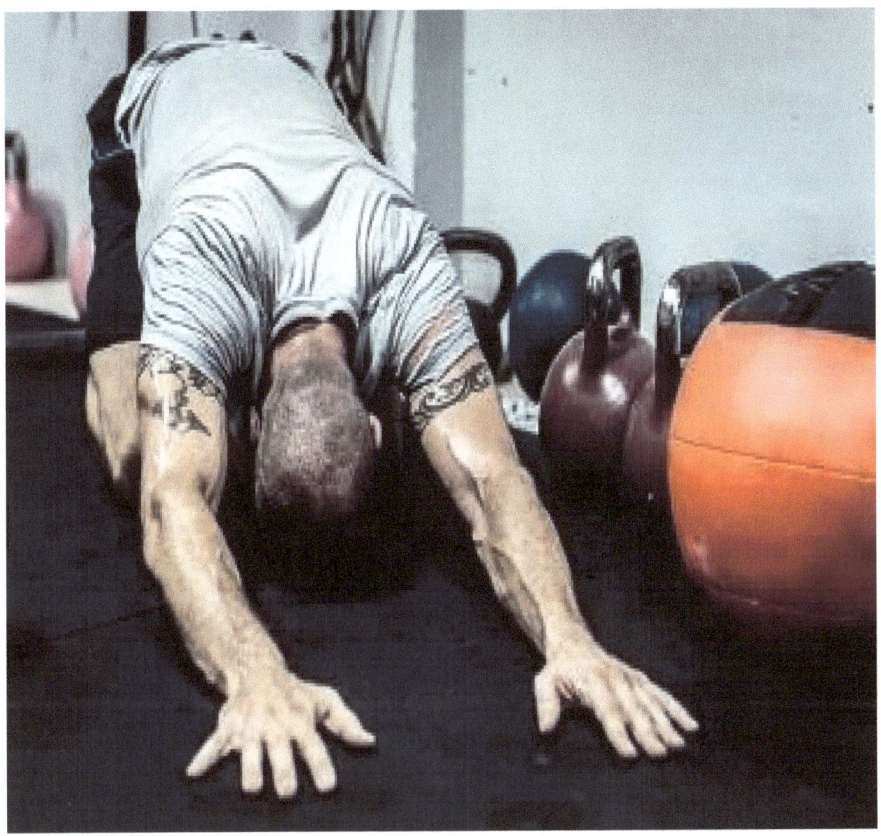

To lose weight and keep trim you need to perform cardio exercises on a regular basis to help to burn more excess fat. This is very important if you want the body of an Alpha Male. The basic rules to losing weight are to lower your calorie intake, and increase the amount of calories you burn.

In general you need to perform 30 - 45 minutes of cardio 3 - 5 times a week to achieve this. There are many exercises that you can perform. Any exercise that increases your heart rate into your target zone and maintains it for 20 minutes or more is considered a cardio exercise. High intensity cardio is the most effective way to lose body fat. If you have a slow metabolism it is even more important to perform cardio exercises.

The best time to perform cardio is in the morning. This is because your carbohydrates are at a minimum at this time in the day. Another good time to carry out cardio exercises is after a weight training session as your body is low on carbs and you will burn body fat for energy. Remember that it is important to perform a mixture of weight training and cardio exercises. Both work great together to help lose body fat, and build muscle.

There are various types of Cardio.

Walking

Walking is a good cardio exercise if you have just started to try and lose weight, or haven't exercised in a while. I try and walk to places if they are not too far away rather than drive or get a taxi. Running / Jogging This type of exercise has high fat burning potential. Early morning or evenings are the best time to perform these exercises. Try running in your local park or around your local streets. Treadmills/ Rowing Machines/ Cross Trainers You can perform a few different types of exercises such as walking, running etc. using these exercise machines.

You can also add resistance to your training and increase the intensity which is great for fat burning. Cycling / Stationary Cycling You can take your mountain bike out for a cycle once in a while. This will give you a break from the gym and you can have fun doing it. Stationary biking is also very good for burning calories. As you perform cardio exercises on a regular basis you will start to find it getting easier. Therefore you need to add resistance to take your cardio respiratory out of its comfort zone.

The Importance of Attitude in a Fitness Program

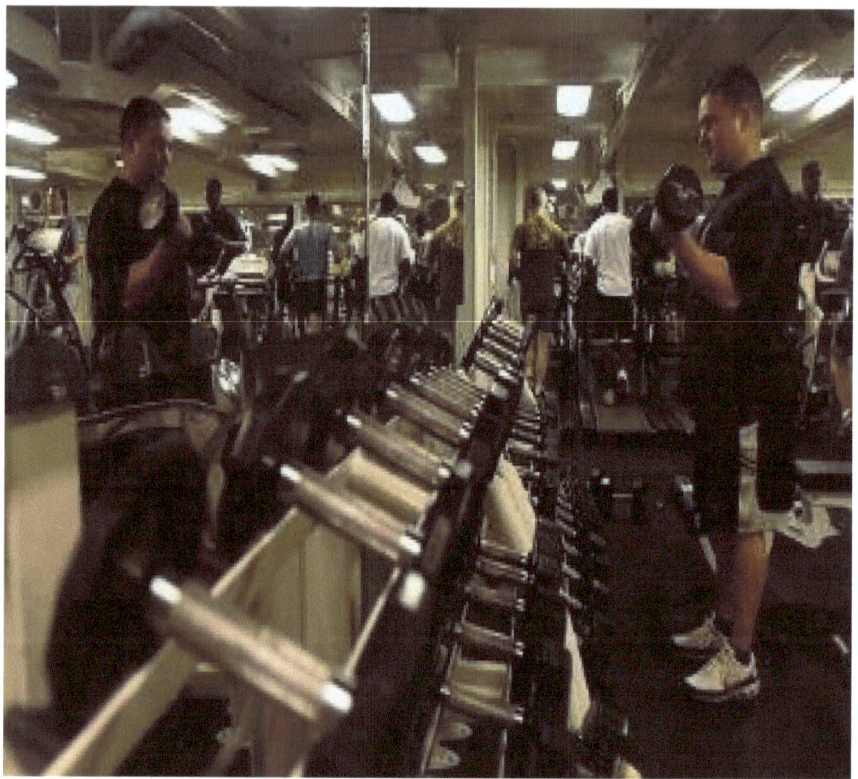

The attitude of a person makes everything attainable. Equal in a lone diet, it is required to hit the right knowledge when it comes to losing weight. This is essential for making you healthy while setting up a diet plan routine. Everything may go wrong if you don't have the right attitude towards your fitness program. Although most diet plans promise you a desirable result afterward, it still won't work if you yourself don't hold on the knowledge of performing it religiously. Even if you're at home, you can do a lot of cardio exercises three to four times a week. This type of exercise allows your heart to work faster preparing for heavier workouts. At normal condition, a heart beats around 60-100 per minute but it increases around 60 - 70% as your heart pumps more oxygenated blood in the body. Although this may take around 20-30 minutes of your regular schedule, this won't apply losing more fat since it doesn't focus into a specific part of the body such as abdominal muscles. Especially if you sign-up a certain fitness program, it is necessary to maintain doing different exercises with a good attitude.

Exercises performed in shaping and building muscles include abdominal workout, biceps and triceps workout, bunk and lessen abdominal exercises, and other bodybuilding exercises. This does not exclude women when we talk some of these exercises. There are also women fitness routine exercises that made specifically for them. Exercises performed are somewhat the same, but sets and repetitions are of great difference. A right attitude in doing these types of exercises is essential if you desire achieving great results. Exercise repetitions can vary according to an individual. You can increase your reps if you're comfortable enough with your current cycle. If you intend to increase the weight, try to lower down your reps for better results. An optimal abs workout can be obtained when exercises are repeatedly done in a day for about 4-5 weeks.

In order for you to prevent workout boredom, you can try doing different exercises since it can help you enhance your will to continue your fitness program till the end. The presence of music can also lighten up your feeling while you're exercising. Attitude in following a proper nutrition should also be regarded along with your fitness program.

Crash dieting is common to those who would want to lose weight in less time, but take note, this is absolutely wrong. A well-balanced diet gives you the right amount of food nutrients necessary for muscle building. The recommended food component ratio goes into 40% protein, 40% carbs, and 20% good fats. Additional nutrients are also important in proper functioning of the body. It is definitely hard to follow a proper diet and good exercise workout especially if you have other things to do. But if you would really like to create a change in your figure, gearing up with the right attitude makes everything possible. A positive attitude does everything to keep you in control, not only during your workout period, but also in everything that you start. Exercise, diet, schedule, repetitions and other components are important in getting a sexy body shape, but attitude of getting it done sounds more essential.

Five Things You Need to Know Now If You Want to Lose Your Gut and Other Unwanted Fat From Your Body

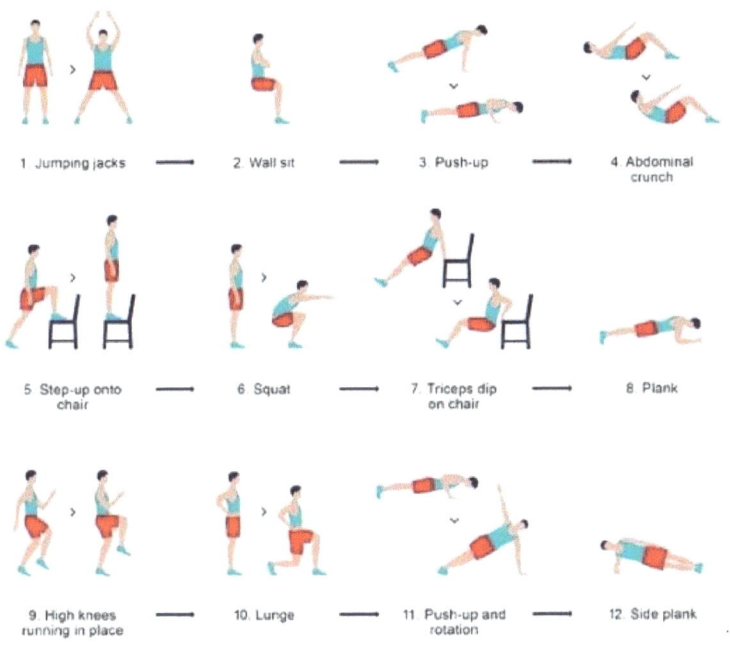

1. Jumping jacks — 2. Wall sit — 3. Push-up — 4. Abdominal crunch

5. Step-up onto chair — 6. Squat — 7. Triceps dip on chair — 8. Plank

9. High knees running in place — 10. Lunge — 11. Push-up and rotation — 12. Side plank

Like many people, I was once young, athletic, and active. I felt like I could eat anything I wanted without concern because my ultra active lifestyle kept me from putting on unwanted pounds. I am 6'2" tall and I was a trim, toned 180 pounds for a long, long time. Then I started a business, and we had a child, then a second, and then a third. I love my job and love my children, but 5 weekly workouts turned into three, then one, then zero. In addition, my kids didn't finish all of their macaroni and cheese. Later, they left behind a chicken nugget. Wow, it had been a long time since I tasted such good food, so a bite here or a nugget there couldn't hurt, right? Well, my 33" pants turned to 34" and later 36" in the waist.

One day, driving home from the zoo with the family, my wife pointed at my growing belly as it protruded over the seat belt in our family hauling minivan and she said, "so how big are you going to let that thing get before you do something about it?". My once flat stomach had become "that thing". What a horrible wake up call. I soon switched to protein bars and nightly sit ups and crunches, waiting for "that thing" to start shrinking. I couldn't wait to get back into my old pants that had slowly worked their way to the bottom of my dresser drawer or the hangars in the back of my closet. However, nothing was working. I humbly realized that I needed guidance and started doing some research.

I soon learned that:

1) Many so-called "health foods" like my protein bars are cleverly disguised junk foods that may actually stimulate more fat production.

2) Crunches, situps, and ab machines are actually some of the least effective exercises for shrinking your gut.

3) Boring repetitive cardio exercises are not necessarily quick ways to lose your gut.

4) Fat burning pills and most powders are a waste of money and many natural foods are more effective and less costly.

5) Most of the ab-belts, ab-rockers, ab-anything that you see on TV are bogus gimmicks and the models on the infomercials never used the products. They obtained their results through real diet and workout plans.

So darn, I couldn't find any shortcuts and I had to really invest some time in figuring out how to do this the right way. I went to a local gym where a trainer tried to sell me on a series of personal training sessions. Oh, this was after going through an embarrassing session of pulling up my shirt for the "before" measurements with a fat caliper.

Driving home after my free first session, I was more sore than I had been in years and I sure didn't want to pay 50 dollars per hour to get killed by a 25 year old who took too much pleasure in what to him seemed like my "old age". You know what I finally did?

I slowed down and took things one step at a time. By learning how to get my diet straightened out by eating more natural foods and COOKING, I started to feel a little better. Then I discovered some really simple exercises focusing on my large muscle groups and my core section, I started to feel a little tighter. Combining this with some realistic and consistent (and moderate) cardio exercises that didn't take more than 20 minutes per day, I actually started to lose the gut, as well as develop some of my old muscle tone. I'm back into a 34" waist on the pants, which works for me and the wife thinks highly of, so I'll be OK if I don't get back to the 33's.

Take your time, save your money, and take things one day at a time, and you too will achieve the results you seek. Also, pick a program that works for you. It's not so much the program as it is getting something that will give you realistic goals so that you can hold yourself accountable. After a while, it becomes a habit and then a lifestyle. You'll feel great and you'll be around longer to enjoy your kids (or grandkids later on). Be smart, be safe, visit my website for more tips, and good luck!

5 Myths to Avoid When Seeking the Best Ab Workout

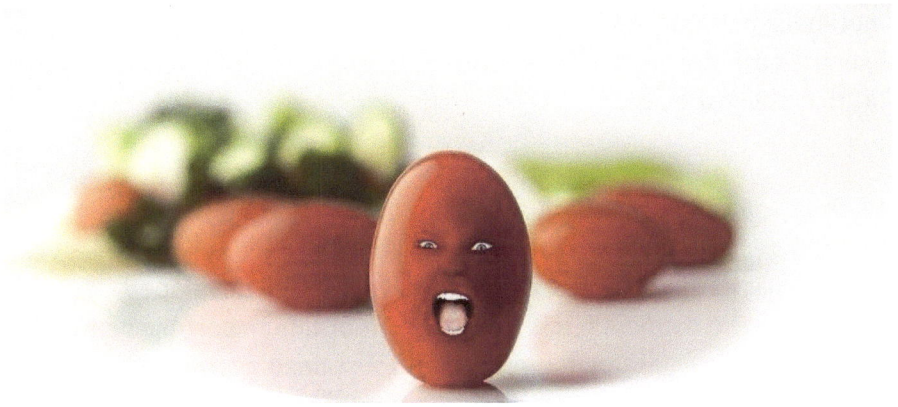

Every day we are bombarded with images of well toned, healthy bodies from ads claiming that we too can have rock hard abs by buying their secret but proven formula. Beyond the hype, good ab workout routines will always involve a proper diet and exercise designed to burn away the layers of body fat that conceal our muscular physique.

So, as we explore all the various diets and workout routines that promise to quickly and easily transform our bodies into the likeness of statuesque Greek gods and goddesses, it's a good idea to be aware of the myths that are sometimes put forward to achieve these goals. Let us start on the right track by exposing the 5 myths that should be avoided.

Myth 1: The best ab workouts require abdominal focused exercises. Truth: The best ab workout routines should focus first on discussing which foods you may be eating that are sabotaging your efforts to lose fat, while promoting the foods that will support a fat burning metabolism. Proper food intake and heart-rate elevated cardio exercises are the most efficient means to reducing the layers of body fat that cover the abs.

Myth 2: You can get six-pack abs in just 10 minutes a day. Truth: Wouldn't everyone have six-pack abs if that were the case? The fact is your six-pack abs will reveal themselves with a well developed nutritional and cardio exercising plan. Your optimum aerobic heart rate zone must be calculated, monitored and sustained over a longer period of time to achieve best results.

Myth 3: You can eliminate problem fat areas with spot fat exercises. Truth: Remember the belt machines that were placed over the belly or butt to vibrate the fat away? We now know that spot fat reduction is simply a myth. While it is true you can develop specific muscle groups with spot training, you cannot burn away fat from specific parts of the body. You must reduce total body fat.

Myth 4: You need to buy equipment like electric contraction belts, sweat suits, ab rockers and twisters to get six-pack abs. Truth: We would all love to have a machine melt away our fat, preferably while we sleep, but the reality is that we need to reduce our overall body fat composition to expose those sought after six-pack abs. Fortunately there are natural fat burning diets along with effective cardio exercises that will help reduce body fat composition faster.

Myth 5: Ab exercises are good cardio exercises. Truth: As stated previously, good cardio exercises require sustaining an elevated heart rate over a given period of time.

You would be better off working your body's larger muscle groups with true cardio exercises like biking, swimming, low impact aerobics, power walking, lunges, squats, sprint runs and resistance or weight training. Focusing on larger muscle groups coupled with a proper diet will burn your fat faster and over a longer period of time. What about pills you ask? Well, many of today's so-called diet pills simply provide a temporary energy boost by stimulating the adrenal glands, which can cause problems with prolonged use.

While most of today's diet pills are ineffectual, there are a few respected researchers doing some promising work in this area. We may well see a pill that mimics aerobic exercise in the future, but as of this writing, these are merely experiments in a lab.

These are some of my other books below, and my website is
www.LosingBellyFatMission.com :

https://www.amazon.com/dp/B06XB4WHZX http://www.amazon.com/dp/B06X9LXBB8
http://www.amazon.com/dp/B06WLK7497

http://www.amazon.com/dp/B06W54JKQN http://www.amazon.com/dp/B06X6DJ9K3
http://www.amazon.com/dp/B06WGNJ9N3 http://www.amazon.com/dp/B06W549TBD
http://www.amazon.com/dp/B06VTF5DQJ http://www.amazon.com/dp/B06WRPSBKK
http://www.amazon.com/dp/B06WD194JR http://www.amazon.com/dp/B06WCZTK7Y
http://www.amazon.com/dp/B06X3QN1HT http://www.amazon.com/dp/B01N19WBF2
http://www.amazon.com/dp/B01N2AVECA http://www.amazon.com/dp/B01N4VZIAV
http://www.amazon.com/dp/B00QJJFS1C http://www.amazon.com/dp/B01EMNO2MW
http://www.amazon.com/dp/B00SSFWCPA http://www.amazon.com/dp/1520531230
http://www.amazon.com/dp/B01N4V7SR9 http://www.amazon.com/dp/B00SX58DUI
http://www.amazon.com/dp/B010K7YP62 http://www.amazon.com/dp/B012LAYNNQ
http://www.amazon.com/dp/B00RVX3KY2 http://www.amazon.com/dp/B01MR6SWGW
http://www.amazon.com/dp/B00XF6G4HO http://www.amazon.com/dp/B01F1472N2
http://www.amazon.com/dp/B00PQ0TUPU http://www.amazon.com/dp/B00PP8OZJ4
http://www.amazon.com/dp/B00QH7DY4Y http://www.amazon.com/dp/B01052010G
http://www.amazon.com/dp/B00QDHXN7Q http://www.amazon.com/dp/B00PO0IQIO

Among others.

www.ingramcontent.com/pod-product-compliance
Lightning Source LLC
Chambersburg PA
CBHW050925290526
45792CB00002B/884